Understanding

FORGETFULNESS
& DEMENTIA

Dr Christopher N. Martyn
& Dr Catharine R. Gale

Published by Family Doctor Publications Limited
in association with the British Medical Association

IMPORTANT NOTICE

This book is intended not as a substitute for personal medical advice but as a supplement to that advice for the patient who wishes to understand more about his/her condition.

Before taking any form of treatment YOU SHOULD ALWAYS CONSULT YOUR MEDICAL PRACTITIONER

In particular (without limit) you should note that advances in medical science occur rapidly and some of the information about drugs and treatment contained in this booklet may very soon be out of date.

© Family Doctor Publications 1995, 1998
Reprinted 1998, 1999

Family Doctor Publications, 10 Butchers Row, Banbury, Oxon OX16 8JH

Medical Editor: Dr Tony Smith
Consultant Editor: Chris McLaughlin
Cover Artist: Dave Eastbury
Illustrations: Angela Christie
Design: MPG Design, Blandford Forum, Dorset
Printing: Reflex Litho, Thetford, Norfolk, using acid-free paper

ISBN: 1-898205-11-6

Contents

I'm worried about my memory   1

How well is your memory working?   8

How to cope with an unreliable memory   12

A sign of something serious?   19

What is dementia?   23

What will your doctor do?   30

The emotional impact   36

Who can help?   41

What can be done?   46

Why did it happen?   49

The future   53

Further reading   56

Useful addresses   57

Index   60

I'm worried about my memory

'I'm always forgetting people's names. Only last week I met someone who used to live just down the road. I knew exactly who she was but I couldn't remember her name. It was so embarrassing. This is happening to me more and more often these days. And I worry about it. Is it going to get worse? Am I getting Alzheimer's disease or going senile?'

This sort of complaint is very common. Many people find that, as they get older, their memory seems to become less and less reliable. Perhaps, like the person speaking above, they meet someone whose face is familiar yet they are quite unable to remember their name.

The problem with memory is often most severe when it comes to

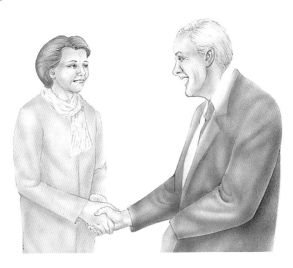

remembering people's names. But someone whose memory for names is unreliable may also be aware of lapses of memory for other things. They may find it difficult to remember appointments, tasks that need to be done, what to buy when out shopping, or where they have put their keys or their spectacles.

When slips of memory occur frequently, it isn't surprising that people become worried. They may come to believe that they are going senile or beginning to develop Alzheimer's disease. While it is true that a deterioration in memory can sometimes be an indication of something serious, there is often a much simpler explanation. If you (or someone close to you) are having trouble remembering things, we hope that the first three chapters in this booklet will help you to understand what is going on, put the problem in a proper perspective and make it easier for you to cope.

How your memory works

Perhaps it would be helpful to start by explaining something about how memory works. Imagine that one morning a friend introduces you to a woman called Muriel Pritchett. Later that day you bump into her again. 'Hello, Muriel,' you say, 'We met this morning.' It is obvious that you have remembered her name. But how?

Despite a great deal of scientific research, there is still much to be learnt about the way memory works, but we already understand quite a lot. One useful way to think about memory is to divide the process into three stages.

Registering new information

The first stage of memory requires that you register the new information. When you were introduced to Muriel, you took note of her name and her face. Your brain absorbs this information and then transfers it to the part where memories are stored.

Storage

During the second stage your brain files away new information. You stored Muriel's name and appearance from the time of your first meeting until you encountered her again.

Recall

The third stage is the retrieval of this information from the part of the brain where it was stored. In our example, this stage occurred when you met Muriel for the second time, and you were able to greet her by name.

All three stages must take place for your memory to work. If any of them had failed, you would have been unable to recall Muriel's name at your second meeting.

In many ways, the process is like putting a letter away in a filing cabinet so that you can refer to it in the future. Think of the letter as the new item of information. First, you have to realise that you may need it again. Second, you must store it in a safe place. And third, when you want to read it again, you have to

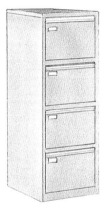

open the right drawer of the filing cabinet and get it out. If you don't notice the importance of the letter in the first place or fail to file it correctly, you won't be able find it when you need it again.

TYPES OF MEMORY

Psychologists believe that there are several different kinds of memory, each of which is used for storing different kinds of information. The part of our memory that we use for

THE THREE STAGES OF MEMORY

- Register new information
- Store this information away
- Retrieve it when needed

storing facts, such as people's names, is separate from the part that we use to store knowledge of how to do things. This explains why some people who have difficulty in remembering names of people they know have no problems remembering how to use a tin-opener or operate a television set.

FORGETTING

We all forget things – indeed, our memory couldn't work properly otherwise. Forgetting can be a useful process in which information that is no longer important is discarded. It wouldn't be sensible to clutter up your brain with memories of everything you bought in the supermarket last week, for example. Your brain makes decisions all the time about what to remember and what to forget. It stores what it considers is important and discards what it thinks is trivial. But every-one's brain makes mistakes from time to time and sometimes things that are significant get forgotten.

All memories tend to fade as

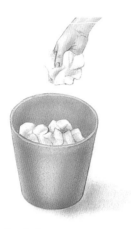

Your brain needs to throw away information to avoid overload.

time passes. Facts used every day stick in the memory while items of information that are seldom needed are harder to recall. For example, most people can remember their own telephone number but, if they need to ring the doctor, they have to look up the number in the phone book.

Recalling a fact or an event keeps that particular memory fresh and makes it easier to remember on future occasions. Conversely, facts that are never used are gradually forgotten. How many dates can you still remember from your history lessons at school?

THINGS THAT INTERFERE WITH MEMORY

The efficiency and accuracy of our memory depend on the circumstances in which we are using it. As we explained earlier, to store a piece of information in the memory, we first have to pay sufficient attention to it to register and absorb it. All sorts of things can interfere with this crucial first stage of memory.

Overload

If we are confronted with too much information at one time, we may find it impossible to recall much of it later. At a social occasion we meet lots of new people, but afterwards it is often difficult to remember their names or much else about them. This is because there was so much information that our capacity to register and store it was overloaded.

People who are very busy may

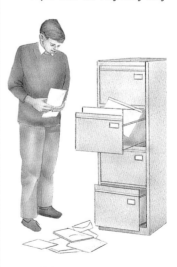

If we are confronted with too much information, we can overload our capacity to register and store it.

find themselves forgetting things simply because they have so much on their minds. If a person's life follows a well-ordered routine, fewer demands are made on their memory than if their life is varied and stressful.

State of mind

For rather similar reasons, people who are anxious or depressed often find that their memory functions poorly. They are preoccupied by their inner feelings and are too distracted by them to pay enough attention to new information to register it properly.

Physical disability

Older people whose hearing or vision is poor may have problems remembering things because their disabilities make it more difficult for them to register and absorb information.

Illness

Physical illness, particularly in older people, can also have a damaging effect on mental function. People who suffer from a chronic condition, such as heart disease or diabetes, may find that their thinking and their memory are not what they were. The reasons for this are not yet well understood, but the stresses of having to cope with illness, especially if the condition is painful, are bound to take their toll.

AGEING IN GENERAL

Every part of the body changes as we get older. Some of these changes begin quite early in life – few athletes and sportsmen continue to break records after the age of 30 or so. Already their muscles, joints, hearts and lungs are performing less well than they were.

Different parts of the body age faster than others, and individuals differ in which parts show the effects of age first. For instance, some people develop osteoarthritis and need a hip replacement, while others become increasingly deaf and have to wear a hearing aid.

AGEING AND MENTAL FUNCTION

It is important to realise that, just as our bodies change as we get older, our mental processes change too. Our reaction time tends to increase and we process new information more slowly. Learning new things is more of a struggle for older people, especially if the information is presented too quickly or in an unfamiliar way. This is because older people tend to find it more difficult to divide their attention between two things at once, and harder to ignore information that is irrelevant to the task in hand. As we get older, we become more concerned with accuracy than speed. This some-times makes us slower when we

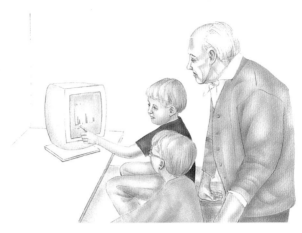

carry out a job. But ageing is not all bad news. Research has shown that older people's greater experience may lead them to develop more efficient ways of doing things, which can outweigh their loss of speed. Indeed, old people often under-estimate their abilities.

HOW MEMORY CHANGES WITH AGE

Psychologists researching how mental function alters as we age have found that there is a gradual change in the way our memory works. One example of this is in the ability to remember a series of numbers for a short period of time. While young people are able to hold a sequence of seven or eight numbers in their heads for a minute or two, most people over the age of 60 or so can only manage to retain a sequence of five or six numbers. You may have noticed this yourself when you have been dialling a telephone number. Our capacity to remember names seems to be especially vulnerable to the effects of age. When it comes to remembering factual information such as what was said in a conversation, the contents of a television programme, or how to do something, most older people manage perfectly well.

Older people who are losing confidence in their ability to remember should take account of the fact that their memories contain much more than the memories of younger people. To go back to an earlier example, their filing cabinets

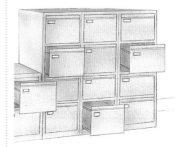

are fuller. At the age of 70, the filing cabinets of memory contain information gathered over a period of time twice as long as those of a person aged 35.

Looked at in this way, it isn't so surprising that older people are slower to retrieve memories and absorb new facts. So, if you are worried about your memory, it makes sense to compare your performance with that of your contemporaries rather than with that of younger people.

KEY POINTS

✓ The memory process can be divided into three stages: registering new information, storage and recall

✓ Everyone forgets things – our brains continually make decisions about what to forget and what to remember

✓ Illness, anxiety and information overload can all affect our ability to remember

✓ Most of us become more forgetful as we grow older

How well is your memory working?

Here is a questionnaire that has been designed to give you an idea of your everyday memory performance. The questions will help you to identify the strengths and weaknesses of your memory.

Find a quiet place and spend a few minutes filling it in. Do try to be as honest as possible.

Each of the questions has four possible answers. These correspond with how often this type of memory lapse happens to you.

Once you have completed the questionnaire, ask someone who lives with you, or a close friend, to make their assessment of how well you remember things. Comparing the score you gave yourself with the score your friend or relative gave you will give you a more realistic view of your memory performance.

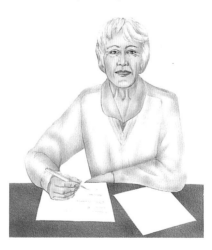

QUESTIONNAIRE

For each question please put a ring around the number which best applies to you. When you have answered all the questions, add up your score.

1 = Never or hardly ever (a few times a year or less)
2 = Occasionally (a few times each month)
3 = Quite often (a few times each week)
4 = Very frequently (every day)

1	Forgetting where you have put something. Losing things around the house	1	(2)	3	4
2	Failing to recognise places that you are told you have often been to before	(1)	2	3	4
3	Having to go back to check whether you have done something that you meant to do	1	2	(3)	4
4	Forgetting to take something with you when you go out	1	2	(3)	4
5	Forgetting that you were told something yesterday or a few days ago, and maybe having to be reminded about it	1	(2)	3	4
6	Failing to recognise, by sight, close relatives or friends whom you meet frequently	(1)	2	3	4
7	When reading a newspaper or magazine; being unable to follow the thread of a story; losing track of what it is about	(1)	(2)	3	4
8	Forgetting to tell somebody something important. Perhaps forgetting to pass on a message or remind someone of something	1	(2)	3	4

continued on page 10

9 Forgetting important details about yourself, for example, your date of birth or where you live	(1)	2	3	4
10 Getting the details of what someone has told you mixed up and confused	1	2	(3)	4
11 Forgetting where things are normally kept or looking for them in the wrong place	(1)	2	3	4
12 Getting lost or turning in the wrong direction on a journey, a walk or in a building where you have OFTEN been before	(1)	2	3	4
13 Doing some routine thing twice by mistake. For example, putting two lots of tea in the teapot, or going to brush your hair when you have just done so	(1)	2	3	4
14 Repeating to someone what you have just told them or asking them the same question twice	1	(2)	3	4
TOTAL SCORE				

We are grateful to Professor Alan Baddeley for allowing us to use an adapted version of his questionnaire on memory lapses.

WHAT DOES YOUR SCORE MEAN

Score	Comments
14–19	Your memory is very good indeed. You have no need to worry
20–29	Your memory performance is about average, but you might find some of the practical advice on memory aids in the next chapter useful
30–39	This score indicates that your memory is below average. This may simply mean that you lead a very busy life, which puts considerable demands on your memory. In the next chapter we give some practical advice on coping with an unreliable memory, which should help you
40–56	This score suggests that your memory is very poor. Frequent memory lapses are likely to have a serious effect on the way you cope with daily life. There may be several reasons for this, but it would be sensible to discuss your memory difficulties with your GP

KEY POINTS

✓ The questionnaire is designed to give you an idea of your everyday memory performance

✓ The questionnaire will help you to identify weaknesses and strengths in your memory function

How to cope with an unreliable memory

Unfortunately your memory is not a system like your heart and lungs for which 'fitness' exercises can be prescribed. Practice at memorising information is very unlikely to improve your memory. Nor is there any evidence that a poor memory can be helped by homeopathic remedies or acupuncture. However, there are a number of things you can do to make life easier, and in this chapter we aim to offer some practical advice on how to cope.

SELF-ASSESSMENT

The first step in coping with a memory that is becoming less reliable is admitting to yourself that you have a problem. The fact that you are reading this book probably indicates that you have taken this step already. We hope that you have tried to answer the questions in the previous chapter. If you have, you should have reached an honest assessment of the state of your memory. It may not be as bad as you had feared.

The second important step is to understand what is happening. As we saw in the first chapter, everyone's memory deteriorates as they get older, and you are not alone in experiencing this problem. Some people prefer to pretend to themselves that nothing is wrong, hoping that their memory problems will go away by themselves, but a positive attitude towards dealing with your difficulties will stand you in much better stead.

BEING HONEST

One extra problem that goes with a failing memory is the embarrassment of forgetting names and faces or letting someone down. In such circumstances, we sometimes try to disguise the fact that we have forgotten in order to save face. After all, it is quite possible to have a chat with someone without saying their name. Or we may try to avoid feelings of awkwardness by joking about our memory lapse, and a sense of humour certainly has its place in coping with the problems of a deteriorating memory.

If your forgetfulness is making life difficult for you, it is tempting to hide your anxiety underneath a joke or to deflect attention from your predicament with a humorous remark, but this tactic may be unwise if it stops you tackling the problem in a serious way. Attempts to disguise the shortcomings of your memory may, in the end, make life more difficult for you.

Why not tell your friends and relatives honestly and straight-forwardly about the difficulties you are having? You will find that others will sympathise – they too will have frequently forgotten people's names, where they put things or tasks they had to do.

FINDING THE RIGHT WORDS

Sometimes it is hard to think of the right words to explain your problems. Try working out a few sentences in advance. Suppose you are worried that you might forget an arrangement to meet a friend. You could say something like 'My memory is becoming rather unreliable – it would help if you could remind me'.

Perhaps you are often faced with the awkward situation of being unable to remember someone's name. Later in this chapter we discuss ways to improve your memory for people's names, but if, despite all your efforts, your mind's still a blank, don't be afraid to admit

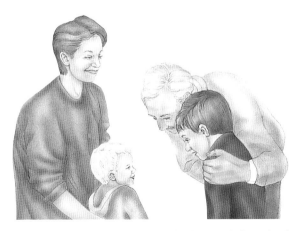

Tell close family members that you are having difficulty remembering so that they can help you.

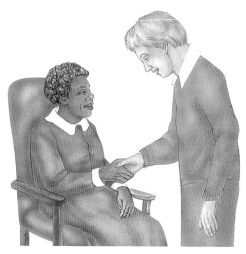

'I remember you very well but I'm afraid I've forgotten your name'

it. Say something like 'I remember you very well, but I'm afraid I've forgotten your name!'.

PRACTICAL WAYS TO COPE

There are a number of practical strategies you can adopt which will help to make memory lapses less frequent. You probably use some memory aids already, such as keeping a diary or making a shopping list, but if you feel that your memory is getting worse, or even if you just wish it were more reliable, it would be sensible to make greater use of them. Relying on such aids reduces the pressure on you to remember and will make you less anxious about forgetting. This in itself may make you less likely to forget things. As we explain later in this chapter, there

are also a number of things that you can do which may improve the way your memory stores information and make it easier to recall it later. Perhaps some of the ideas we recommend will seem too simple to be of much use, but do give them a try anyway. Lots of people whose memories have been letting them down have found them surprisingly helpful.

MEMORY PROMPT FOR TASKS

If you find that you are forgetting things you have to do, try using some of the following memory prompts.

Notes

Written notes are a simple but very effective reminder. Keep a notebook

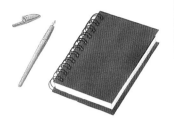

with you during the day so you can write down all your tasks, particularly those that you can't do immediately. These are the ones that you are most likely to forget. Try to get into the habit of making a note as soon as you think of something that you've got to do. Look at your notebook regularly, perhaps two or three times a day – there is no point writing reminders to yourself unless you are going to see them frequently. Some people find that, when they are in bed at night, they remember things they need to do the next day. It's a good idea to keep a paper and pen by your bed so you can jot down these ideas when they occur to you.

Another way of prompting yourself is to stick up a note in a place where you cannot fail to see it. Stationers sell brightly coloured pads of sticky paper called 'Post-it'

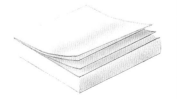

notes, specially designed for leaving notes for yourself or other people. These are particularly useful if you have problems remembering to do something. For instance, if you need to take your coat to the cleaners, you could stick a note to yourself on the front door.

Diaries and wall-calendars

Diaries or wall-calendars are also useful ways of reminding yourself to do things. Get into the habit of writing down all your appointments and all the things that you need to do on a particular day. Put your diary or calendar somewhere – the hall or the kitchen – where you will see it several times a day.

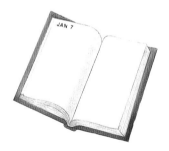

Lists

Most people make shopping lists, especially when they have a lot to buy, but they can be useful at other times too. For instance, it can be helpful to make a list of things that you need to talk about before you telephone someone.

When you are planning to go

away on holiday, make a list of everything that you need to pack, tick each item off as you pack it, and take a final look at the list again before you leave home.

Tablet organisers

If you need to remember to do something regularly, such as taking tablets, why not buy the type of watch that can give an alarm at set times. Alternatively, you could opt for a special pill box with an alarm, or one that's divided into compartments for each day of the week to make it much easier to remember to take your daily dose and check that you have taken it.

Another way of remembering is to keep the tablets near to something you use at about the time you should take them. For example, you could put the bottle of tablets next to your toothbrush or the tea caddy. Having an established routine puts

less stress on your memory, and you may find that, if you regularly do things in a set order, you will do them almost automatically.

IMPROVING YOUR MEMORY FOR TASKS

On page 2, we explained how items of information are properly stored in your memory if you pay attention to them. If you get into the habit of regularly thinking about the things that you have to do, you are more likely to remember them. You may find it helpful to think about what you have to do at set times of the day, such as when you start work or after lunch. This rehearsal of tasks helps to keep them in your mind.

Sometimes you may find that you know there is something that you need to do but you cannot remember exactly what it was. In this situation, it can often help to go

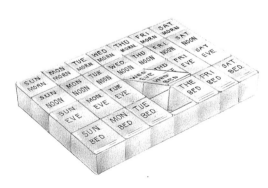

A medicine dispenser is invaluable to remind you when to take your medication.

over other things that you had to do to try to prompt your memory. For example, if you are out shopping, you could think about all the other things that you meant to buy. Or suppose there is some job in the garden you planned to do, but you have forgotten what it was – try casting your mind back to when you first thought about this particular task, or go out to the garden. Either of these actions will help to stimulate your memory.

People often forget whether or not they have done a particular thing, such as shutting a window or turning off the oven. One way to help yourself remember is to talk out loud about what you are doing as you do it. So, when you turn the oven off say 'I'm turning the oven off now'. This concentrates your mind on what you are doing and helps to fix it in your memory.

TIPS FOR FINDING THINGS

It is all too easy to put our glasses or keys down somewhere and then be unable to find them later. Or perhaps we buy something, put it away and forget where it is.

Organisation
Being well organised and keeping things in set places can help. Try to put things away in their proper place after you've used them. If you tend to mislay your keys around the house, you could put up a special

hook for them and get into the habit of hanging them there as soon as you come into the house.

Lists and labels
It may also help to write down a list of where you usually keep things, and use it to ensure that you put things away in the right place. Labelling cupboards with a list of the contents is a good idea too.

Self-adhesive labels with your name, address and telephone number are also useful if you have a tendency to leave things behind when you are out. Stick them on possessions like your umbrella or bag, then, if you do forget them, at least someone can return them to you.

Remembering where you put something
When you put something away, make a deliberate effort to concen-

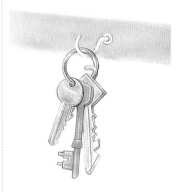

A place for everything and everything in its place.

trate on the particular place where you are putting it. Is there a reason why you are putting it in that particular place? You may find that saying out loud where you are putting something as you do it helps to fix it in your memory. Forming a connection between the object and the place where you are putting it also helps you to remember it later.

For example, when you park your car in a car park, concentrate on the position of the car in relation to a ticket machine or the exit. After you have walked away from the car, picturing it and its position in the car park will help to store the memory properly.

If you do forget where you put something, go back in your mind to when you last remember having it. What were you doing? Then think what you did next and where you were. Alternatively, think of all the places where you're likely to have put it.

REMEMBERING NAMES

When you meet someone for the first time, pay close attention to their name. If it's an unusual one, ask how it is spelt. As you talk to them, use their name – 'Where do you live, Muriel?'. Repeating someone's name in conversation is a friendly thing to do and, the more attention you pay to their name, the more likely it is to become fixed in your memory. When you say goodbye, say their name again.

If someone's name is on the tip of your tongue, try going through the alphabet letter by letter. If possible, think back to where you first heard their name. This might help you remember but, if you still can't recall their name, don't be afraid to admit it. This is a very common problem!

KEY POINTS

✓ Admitting that you have a problem is the first step to coping with an unreliable memory

✓ Tell your friends and family that you are having difficulty with your memory

✓ To help you remember where things are, decide on a particular place for articles that you frequently mislay, and label cupboards and drawers

A sign of something serious?

Many people who find that their memories are beginning to let them down worry that they are developing a serious disease of the brain. They may harbour the suspicion that they are becoming senile or are developing Alzheimer's disease. Indeed, for some people, this is the worst aspect of a failing memory. The inconvenience and embarrassment that result from a poor memory may worry them far less than the fear that their increasing memory lapses are a symptom of senility or dementia. They feel that they could cope with their memory problems as long as they knew that they were not going to become demented.

In the first part of this booklet, we described the normal changes in memory capacity that happen as we get older. We tried to be reassuring and point out that an increasing number of memory lapses are simply something you have to learn to live with. But sometimes changes in mental function are a sign that something more serious than simple ageing is happening to the brain, and in the next few pages we discuss the sort of things that you or the person you are worried about should take along to your doctor.

CASE HISTORY: DEMENTIA

Ralph Emerson retired from his job at the town hall a few months before his 65th birthday. At first, he and his wife, Lydia, had been busy doing all the things they had always promised themselves that they would do when they had time. Ralph redecorated the house and Lydia made new curtains. They kept fit by going swimming twice each week and took up new hobbies. Lydia discovered that she had a talent for painting in water colours and Ralph taught himself to make

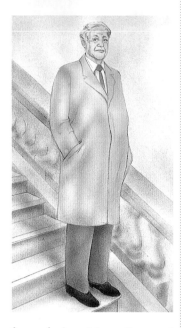

frames for her pictures. They went off on holiday to places that they had always wanted to visit and, one winter, they went to visit their eldest daughter and her family in Australia. For a few years Lydia thought that she had never known Ralph so happy. Gradually, however, she became aware that he wasn't quite his usual self.

Since retirement, it had become Ralph's habit to do the weekly shopping. Lydia had been delighted to have someone take over a chore that she had never much liked. Ralph rather enjoyed it, taking a pride in getting the best value for money and showing off his bargains with schoolboy pleasure to his wife when he returned. But, over the past months, he seemed to have become a spendthrift.

On several occasions he had come home with too many vegetables and expensive cuts of meat that were too big for the two of them to eat. Once he had bought tins of pet food – and they didn't even have a cat or dog. Ralph also began to forget things although Lydia had given him a shopping list.

Lydia decided that she needed to go to the supermarket with him. They did their shopping and queued up at the checkout. When it was time to pay, Ralph got out his wallet. But he looked unsure what to do next. Lydia was horrified to see that Ralph couldn't work out how much money to give the woman at the till. She had to take over and count out the notes herself.

Ralph began to change in other ways too. He had always been a good-natured man even when he had been under pressure at work, but now, it seemed to Lydia, he was often moody and bad tempered.

Little things seemed to upset him and he reacted to minor irritations with uncharacteristic outbursts of bad language. Some of their friends commented on the change in Ralph's personality too, so she knew it wasn't just her imagination.

As time went on, Lydia got more and more worried about her

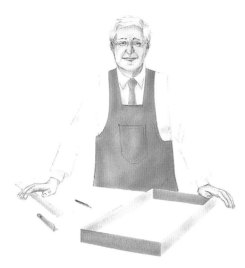

husband. Tasks that he had previously accomplished without difficulty were now beyond him, and he no longer had the ability to concentrate on anything for any length of time.

When he tried to make a frame for a picture that Lydia had painted, it turned out the wrong size. And absurdly he blamed Lydia for using too large a piece of paper rather than himself for not measuring accurately.

Lydia also noticed that he had completely run out of energy and drive. He no longer suggested going on outings to do the sort of things that they had so enjoyed together in the past. Indeed, he didn't really like leaving the house, and Lydia suspected that he became frightened and bewildered as soon as he was any distance from home. Several times neighbours had found him apparently lost in a nearby street and had to lead him home.

Even at home he showed little interest in what was going on. He appeared to read the newspaper over breakfast as he had always

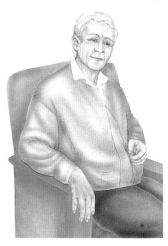

done, but she noticed that later in the day he had no recollection of any of the headlines. When old friends came to visit, he took little part in the conversation. Sometimes, in fact, he didn't even seem to know who they were.

Ralph's dementia began at an unusually young age – it is rare in people under the age of 70. But his decline illustrates many of the changes in personality and mental function that are common in the early stages of this disease. It also shows the striking difference between the very common memory lapses that come with ageing and the devastating impact of dementia.

Memory lapses are embarrassing and a nuisance, but the individual's personality and ability to solve the problems of everyday life remain the same. Dementia is quite different. Ralph's symptoms have been brought about by disease, which causes a deterioration in almost every aspect of brain function.

KEY POINTS

✓ People often worry that memory problems are a sign of dementia

✓ Most memory lapses are not caused by dementia

✓ Dementia is a disease that affects personality and the ability to cope with everyday life

What is dementia?

Dementia is a term used by doctors to describe a progressive deterioration in mental powers accompanied by changes in behaviour and personality.

The story we told about Ralph in the last chapter illustrates some of the changes that are most frequently seen in someone who is suffering from the early stages of dementia. Individuals, of course, differ in the way that they respond to a disease. Depending on their age, the sort of person they are and their physical health, the symptoms may vary a little between one person and another.

WHAT ARE THE SYMPTOMS OF DEMENTIA?

The symptoms of dementia include memory loss, personality changes, disorientation, inability to perform daily routine activities and difficulty in communication.

Memory loss

This is a common feature of dementia, and the memory for recent events is affected first. The capacity to remember further back in time usually remains unaffected until the disease is at a more advanced stage. The ability to store recent information deteriorates because of the changes in the brain that occur in diseases such as Alzheimer's. In the early stages, this problem with short-term memory may not create too many difficulties; after all, many people find that their memories are less good as they get older. But, as the disease progresses, memory loss will become more severe. Sufferers may set out on an errand, for example, and then forget where they were going, or they may have a meal and later forget that they have eaten. In the later stages, they may even forget the names of people close to them.

THE MOST COMMON PROBLEMS OF DEMENTIA

- Deterioration of memory
- Disorientation
- Changes in personality and behaviour
- Loss of practical everyday skills
- Difficulty in communicating

Disorientation

Closely connected to the failure of memory is the loss of the ability to orientate oneself in direction or time. Many sufferers from dementia show signs of being disorientated, not knowing where they are or the correct year, month or day of the week. Sometimes they may get day and night muddled up, wanting to go out in the middle of the night or sleep during the day. You will remember from the last chapter how Ralph appeared bewildered when he was any distance from home. This deterioration in the ability to find one's way around becomes more marked as the disease advances. Sufferers may become more likely to wander away from home and get lost, which can pose a particular problem for those caring for them. In the later stages of the illness, they may have problems finding their way around their own home.

Personality and behaviour

Some sufferers' personalities seem to remain much as they were before the onset of the disease, but others may show quite striking changes. Social withdrawal and a loss of interest in usual activities are common. People with dementia may experience uncharacteristic mood swings, or some underlying part of their personality may become much more pronounced. They may develop a tendency to spitefulness or anxiety, for example. Some people seem to undergo drastic alterations in personality, changing perhaps from being gentle and placid most of the time into a person prone to outbursts of temper and aggression.

As the disease progresses, many sufferers start to behave in ways that are socially unacceptable, and may do or say things that would once have seemed quite inappropriate for them.

Loss of practical skills

In the last chapter we saw how Ralph lost the ability to accomplish everyday tasks and how he found it hard to concentrate on anything for any length of time. This is one of the features of dementia. Sufferers have difficulty in performing actions that

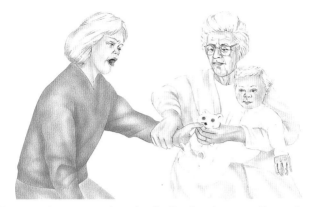

Some people seem to undergo drastic alterations in personality – perhaps prone to outbursts of temper and aggression.

they used to manage easily, such as driving a car, cooking and, as the disease gets worse, even dressing or washing themselves.

Difficulty in communication

In the early stages of dementia people may have difficulty in finding the correct word to use when they are speaking. This makes it harder for them to engage in complicated conversations, and taking down messages over the telephone can be a particular problem.

Later, they may be unable to finish sentences, wandering off on to another subject, or they may repeat words over and over again. The ability to read and write may also be affected.

It becomes more difficult to find the right word when speaking as the disease progresses and, as powers of comprehension also decline, conversation becomes increasingly harder.

Non-verbal forms of communication, such as touch and expression, become very important for those caring for people in the later stages of dementia.

WHAT CAUSES DEMENTIA?

The medical label of dementia doesn't amount to a complete diagnosis. A number of separate diseases can produce the symptoms of dementia and it is important to find out which of these is the cause.

Some can be treated successfully although, unfortunately, there are others about which little can be done at the moment.

Alzheimer's disease

Alzheimer's disease is the most common cause of dementia in

POSSIBLE CAUSES

- Alzheimer's disease
- Stroke or vascular dementia
- Vitamin B_{12} deficiency
- Underactive thyroid
- Drug interactions
- Hereditary diseases of the nervous system
- Delayed effects of repeated head injury

elderly people living in the UK. In a very few cases the disease occurs because of a defective gene. The gene is inherited, so several members of the same family may be affected. We must emphasise, however, that this is an unusual reason for developing Alzheimer's disease, and most cases are not caused by this genetic abnormality. Scientists have not yet discovered the cause for the much more common form of this condition, which does not run in families. An enormous amount of research is being devoted to Alzheimer's disease at the moment, and some of the recent advances and current theories are described on pages 51–2.

Scientists have also been studying what happens to the nerve cells in the brains of sufferers. When

a powerful microscope is used to look at a thin slice of brain from a patient with Alzheimer's disease at high magnification, two unusual features, not present in the brains of normal people, can be seen. These features are called senile plaques and neurofibrillary tangles. The plaque is an accumulation of an abnormal protein called amyloid. One theory of Alzheimer's disease suggests that this plaque forms because the processes that normally operate to clear away this protein have become defective. Neurofibrillary tangles are skeins of another abnormal protein but, unlike the senile plaque, the tangle is found inside the nerve cells. The reason why these tangles develop is not properly understood, but once again it seems that the normal processing of protein by the cell is disrupted in some way. These tangles choke up the nerve cells and prevent them from working properly.

Vascular dementia

Almost every part of the body needs to be supplied with blood – it carries oxygen and nutrients to the tissues and takes away carbon dioxide and other waste products of metabolism – and the brain is no exception. It is a very active organ and is richly supplied with blood through a dense network of many millions of tiny blood vessels.

If some of these tiny blood vessels become blocked, they can no longer carry out their function of delivering blood. This is what happens when someone has a mild stroke. The areas of the brain that they previously supplied become short of oxygen, and some of the nerve cells die. An area of tissue that has died because of lack of oxygen is called an infarct.

Widespread disease of the small blood vessels can lead to the appearance of many tiny infarcts throughout the substance of the brain. It is not too hard to understand that, although each individual infarct is very small, the cumulative effect of many infarcts will disrupt normal brain function. Sometimes this form of dementia is called multi-infarct dementia.

Our blood vessels tend to get narrower as we get older. The process is a little like the furring up of pipes and kettles that occurs in hard water areas of the country. However, disease of small blood vessels is particularly common in people who have had high blood pressure for a long period of time, and it may be made worse by smoking cigarettes.

Mixed dementia

Sometimes, when the brain of a person who has died from dementia is examined, features of

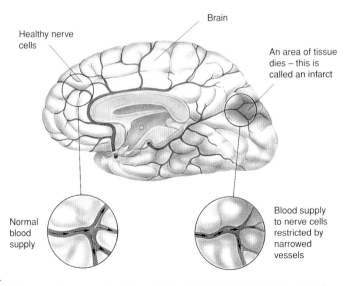

The brain needs a rich supply of blood. If the supply is restricted or blocked, some of the cells may die – this is called an infarct.

Alzheimer's disease and many tiny infarcts are found. It may be impossible to decide whether the patient's symptoms were caused by Alzheimer's disease or vascular dementia, so such people are said to have suffered from a mixed dementia.

Other causes of dementia

The list of causes in the box on page 26 shows that dementia can occur for many reasons.

Sometimes the symptoms of dementia arise because of a metabolic or hormonal disturbance. For example, vitamin B_{12} deficiency, an underactive thyroid or, rarely, an adverse reaction to drug treatments can upset the balance of salts and chemicals in the blood and brain. If the dementia is caused by something like this, it can usually be treated successfully.

There are a large number of hereditary diseases that can also cause dementia. Fortunately these are all very rare.

Repeated head injuries, such as those suffered by professional boxers, sometimes result in the later development of a form of dementia.

If you want to find out more about Alzheimer's disease, vascular dementia or the other rare causes of dementia, turn to page 56 where we recommend some books that you may find helpful.

WHAT SHOULD YOU DO?

If you are concerned that someone close to you is showing symptoms similar to those just described, you should seek medical advice. There are several reasons why you should take action sooner rather than later. First, it can be quite difficult to diagnose dementia correctly. The symptoms that are worrying you may have another explanation. One illness that often produces symptoms very similar to dementia, particularly in elderly people, is depression. You probably think of depression in terms of feeling low in spirits and pessimistic about the future, but clinical depression means much more than the temporary gloominess that we all feel occasionally. People suffering from severe depression may show so much difficulty with memory and concentration and loss of interest in their surroundings that they appear to be suffering from dementia.

A second reason for talking to your doctor is that some illnesses that produce symptoms of dementia can be cured and it is important to diagnose these as early as possible. Even if the condition is incurable, treatment may be available that will stop the symptoms getting worse. Last, if it does turn out to be a form of dementia for which there is no treatment, there is still much that can be offered in the way of practical help and support to improve the quality of life of the sufferer, and to ease the burden of those who care for them.

KEY POINTS

✓ The symptoms of dementia include severe memory problems, disorientation, difficulties in communication, personality changes and alterations in usual behaviour

✓ Dementia can arise by a number of different causes, the most common of which are Alzheimer's disease and vascular dementia

✓ Medical help should be sought as soon as possible

What will your doctor do?

The previous chapter ended with the advice that, if you are worried about your own mental function or are concerned that someone close to you is developing signs of becoming demented, you should consult your GP right away. Here we explain how your doctor is likely to approach the problem, following Ralph and Lydia's story as an example. This will help you to be prepared for the questions that you will be asked. We also describe briefly some of the tests that your doctor may feel are necessary and explain the reason for doing them.

THE MEDICAL HISTORY

Let us imagine that Lydia has persuaded Ralph to consult his doctor. They make an appointment to see his GP, Dr Elizabeth Garrett, and Lydia is going with her husband. To make a diagnosis Dr Garrett will need a detailed account

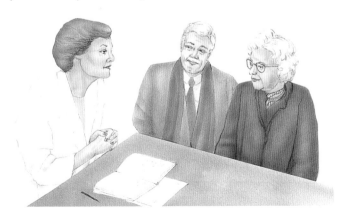

of what has been happening to Ralph over the past months. Since Ralph is often rather muddled, it will be up to Lydia to provide reliable information. Although people often think that doctors make their diagnoses from the results of scientific tests like X-rays or laboratory blood tests, the first and most crucial step is actually obtaining a clear description of the illness from the patient or a reliable witness. Tests come later and are used to confirm the doctor's clinical judgement or to help distinguish between a small number of possible causes of the illness. Lydia's story of the changes that have occurred in Ralph will be the first and most important clue in finding out what is wrong. By talking to Lydia as well as Ralph, Dr Garrett will gain a fuller picture of the situation.

Dr Garrett will want to know:

- whether any members of Ralph's family have suffered from a disease of the nervous system
- details of Ralph's past illnesses, if any, although she may well have a record of this
- whether Ralph is taking any medication, either prescribed for him by a doctor or medicines that he has bought for himself at the chemist. Sometimes the wrong dose of a drug or a mixture of drugs taken together can produced a confused state of mind that resembles dementia.

Dr Garrett will also probably:

- measure his blood pressure
- carry out a physical examination, paying particular attention to the function of the nervous system
- perform various tests of mental performance. These won't be alarming, but will allow her to assess Ralph's memory and problem-solving abilities, so that she can confirm Lydia's story and assess the extent of Ralph's mental deterioration.

Depending on what Dr Garrett finds, she may arrange for some tests to be done herself or she may want to arrange for Ralph to see a specialist who has expert knowledge and experience of dementia and its associated problems.

SPECIALISTS

The availability of specialists varies from one part of the country to another. The type of specialist to whom a GP refers a patient with suspected dementia will depend partly on what services are available in that particular area, but also on the characteristics of the patients, such as their age and the nature of their symptoms.

The clinical psychologist

It is often helpful if a clinical psychologist assesses someone with suspected dementia as he or she is trained to assess memory, learning ability and other mental functions. During an interview lasting about an hour, he or she will administer a number of tests. The results will provide a more detailed picture of a patient's mental abilities and difficulties.

The neurologist

Neurologists are doctors who specialise in seeing patients with disorders of the brain and other parts of the nervous system. They look after patients with conditions such as Parkinson's disease, epilepsy, multiple sclerosis and migraine. These patients frequently need brain scans and other tests that can be done only using expensive machines. For this reason neurologists tend to work in the larger hospitals that contain such equipment.

If Dr Garrett suspects that Ralph's symptoms are caused by a disease of the brain, she might consider referring him to a neurologist for a specialist opinion and, if necessary, further investigation.

The geriatrician

Geriatricians specialise in the diseases and illnesses of elderly people. Failure of memory and deterioration of mental function are, of course, quite common in older people, and geriatricians are expert at investigating to find out the underlying reason for these mental changes. Older people are often reluctant to go to hospital, and so geriatricians often visit patients at home to assess and examine them there.

Geriatricians often work as part of a team made up of nurses, occupational therapists, physio-therapists and social workers, and they have particular expertise in arranging support for elderly people living at home.

The psychiatrist

Psychiatrists are doctors who specialise in diagnosing and treating a wide range of mental health problems. Their assessment can be particularly helpful in cases where severe depression may be causing symptoms similar to those of dementia.

The psychogeriatrician

A psychogeriatrician is a psychiatrist who specialises in the mental health problems of elderly people. They have a great deal of experience in diagnosing dementia, in advising on the problems associated with the disease and in coordinating medical and social services to help look after sufferers.

TESTS AND INVESTIGATIONS

There are a number of tests available designed primarily to exclude other possible causes of mental malfunction such as hormone dysfunction, chest infection, heart or lung disorder or a brain tumour.

Blood tests

Sometimes a deterioration in mental functioning can be a result of a disturbance in the body's metabolism or an imbalance in the hormones circulating in the bloodstream. Analysis of a specimen of blood in the laboratory allows such a disturbance or imbalance to be detected. The laboratory analysis may be tricky because accurate measurements have to be made of very tiny amounts of chemicals and hormones, and it sometimes takes a week or two before the results are sent back to the doctor who requested the tests. But, from the patient's point of view, these tests are easy and nearly painless. A small amount of blood is removed from a vein at the elbow or in the back of the hand. It is stored in a special tube until the laboratory is ready to carry out the analysis. All the patient has to do is wait for the answer.

X-rays

X-rays of the chest may be carried out to see if a chest infection or some disorder of the heart or lungs is contributing to the deterioration in mental function.

CT

The letters CT stand for computed tomography – a sophisticated type of X-ray that allows the brain to be visualised in great detail. The person whose brain is being scanned lies on a table with the head inside a large circular hole,

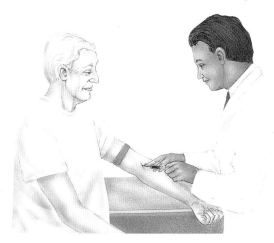

Taking a blood test.

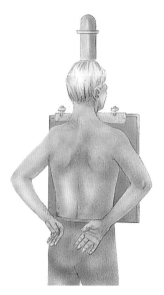

Having a chest X-ray.

positions, enabling the doctor to see whether there are any abnormalities that might be causing the symptoms.

WHAT WILL HAPPEN NEXT?

Once all the necessary tests and investigations have been carried out, the results will be sent to Dr Garrett. If she referred Ralph to a specialist, they will write to her, giving her the results of any investigations they carried out, their assessment of his condition, and perhaps recommendations about treatment. It may take several months and perhaps several hospital visits before a definite diagnosis can be made. There is no simple test to show whether a person is suffering from a progressive form of dementia, such as Alzheimer's disease. This

around which is the scanning machinery. The scanner produces a series of pictures showing cross-sections of the brain at different

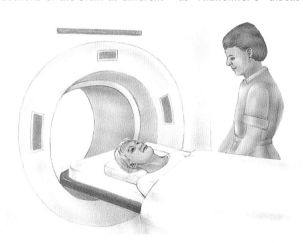

Undergoing a CT scan.

diagnosis can be made only when other possible causes of the symptoms have been eliminated.

When the tests and assessments have been completed, Lydia and Ralph will be able to go back either to Dr Garrett or to the hospital specialist to discuss the results and plan how Ralph's problems should be dealt with.

KEY POINTS

✓ The carer of a person suspected of dementia will be asked about the patient's recent behaviour

✓ The doctor will perform a physical examination and a number of mental performance tests to help him or her to make a diagnosis

✓ The patient may be referred for specialist help

The emotional impact

Coming to terms with the fact that a member of your family is suffering from a progressive form of dementia, such as Alzheimer's disease, is very difficult. It is hard enough in the early stages to cope with the shock of the diagnosis and the changes that are already noticeable in the sufferer. As the patient's illness progresses and the symptoms worsen, you will have to adjust to new signs of deterioration. People who care for someone with a chronic, dementing illness need a great deal of support to help them deal with the powerful emotions that their sad predicament is bound to produce. It is very important, if you are in such a position, to recognise your own feelings and to realise that you will need emotional support from others. Far from being selfish, this will help you to cope more effectively.

In this chapter we describe some of the feelings that you may experience and offer some advice.

SENSE OF LOSS

When someone close to you is diagnosed as suffering from dementia, you are bound to feel grief. The changes that the disease brings about in the sufferer's personality and behaviour and their increasing inability to live a normal life arouse emotions similar to those experienced after a bereavement. You will have to cope with feelings of sadness and distress at the loss of companionship – you are losing someone with whom you previously shared concerns and joys and you may also be losing a sexual partner. This sense of grief will be heightened as you gradually understand the implications of the diagnosis. Coming to terms with your own feelings at the same time as having to look after the sufferer is a double burden.

What should you do? Sharing your concerns and feelings with family and friends can help you accept the situation and perhaps ease the sense of loss. Your doctor will be able to offer you psychological support and to refer you for counselling if you think this would help. Meeting other people who are in a similar situation is another way of finding this sort of psychological help.

There are support groups for carers in most parts of the country and there should be one near you. Some of these are independent local carers' groups, while others are run by national organisations. The Alzheimer's Disease Society specialises in the needs of carers looking after people with all kinds of dementia. Age Concern and the Carers National Association are also involved in support groups for the carers of dementia sufferers. The last chapter of this book contains addresses and telephone numbers of these organisations. If there is no support group in your area, perhaps you could start one. Your doctor or district nurse will probably be able to put you in touch with other families, and you could put up a notice in your local surgery or library asking people who are interested to contact you.

ANGER

It is natural to feel angry and resentful: angry that such a terrible thing has happened, angry perhaps that other members of the family don't help enough, and resentful that the future you had looked forward to has changed. In addition, you will have to deal with the daily exasperations and irritations of looking after the sufferer. People

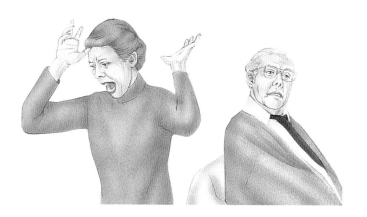

It is natural for a carer to feel anger and frustration from time to time.

with dementia behave in ways that may make them very hard to live with.

Many people fail to recognise their anger or are frightened to express it. They may pretend to themselves that they are not really angry. Perhaps they are ashamed that they are angry with someone who is ill. But denying or bottling up these feelings of anger is not a good idea. Unless it is recognised and expressed, anger will lead to bitterness and resentment, and this will only make it harder to cope with daily life.

One way of handling these feelings is to find ways to express them. Talk to other people about your irritation and anger. Other carers will know what you are going through, and discussing your feelings with them will help you to cope better.

GUILT

Guilt is also a common emotional reaction. When the disease is first diagnosed, it is natural to look for some explanation for what has happened. Sometimes people feel that perhaps something they did or failed to do caused the illness. If you have worries like this, it may be helpful to learn more about the disease and to discuss your concerns with your doctor.

Feeling embarrassed or even disgusted by the sufferer's behav-

COMMON EMOTIONAL REACTIONS EXPERIENCED BY CARERS

- Sense of loss
- Feelings of anger
- Guilt
- Embarrassment
- Loneliness

iour, losing your temper, wishing someone else could take on the responsibility of caring, or caring for someone to whom one has never been close – all these can produce feelings of guilt.

You may feel resentful and uncomfortable at having to take on tasks that were normally the responsibility of the sufferer, and this too can cause guilt feelings. Caring for someone with dementia can sometimes involve a reversal of roles. You may be in a position of behaving like a parent to your mother or father. The sort of assistance that sufferers need is that required by a small child from his or her parents, such as help with feeding and washing. It can be hard to adjust to this change of roles.

Most of us find it hard to accept that we cannot always live up to the expectations of ourselves or others. It is very important to be aware of your feelings, to try to appraise the situation realistically and not to expect too much from yourself. You may reach a stage when you feel that the difficulties and stresses that caring for a demented person impose on you and other family members are too great, and that the time has come to arrange for long-term residential care for the sufferer. This decision may produce a sense of relief as the burden is lifted, but also intense feelings of guilt. Talking things over with others may help. Realising that such feelings are common and discussing how other people have coped with them will help keep your guilt feelings in their proper perspective.

EMBARRASSMENT

One of the early effects of dementia is a loss of sensitivity to other people in social situations. The skills that are needed to maintain relationships are often among the first to disappear. The sufferer may lose the judgement necessary to behave or speak appropriately. It may become embarrassing to take them out, especially as strangers often do not understand what is happening. One way of dealing with this is to share your experiences with other carers.

Learning how others manage will help you to handle such problems with greater aplomb and less embarrassment, and even to laugh about them. Explaining the illness to neighbours and friends can also reduce your embarrassment, as they will then understand the reason for the sufferer's behaviour.

LONELINESS

Being a carer is a lonely experience. The pressures of looking after a demented person make it difficult to maintain social activities. You may feel very much alone if the sufferer is the person with whom you used to share everything. Loneliness can make it harder to solve the problems of everyday life, so it is important not to let caring for the sufferer prevent you devoting time to your own needs. Make arrangements to share the care so you can spend time with family and friends or go to meetings and support groups for carers, such as those run by the Alzheimer's Disease Society. Talking to other people in a similar situation, who understand your feelings, can provide both support and friendship. Make some time for yourself to do things that you enjoy.

KEY POINTS

✓ It is extremely difficult to come to terms with the fact that someone close to you is deteriorating mentally

✓ Emotional reactions to the diagnosis of dementia include a sense of loss, and feelings of anger, guilt, embarrassment and loneliness

Who can help?

If you are caring for someone with dementia, you are likely to need a good deal of practical support. The sufferer will find it increasingly hard to cope with everyday life, and you will not be able to provide all the assistance that they need without help. Unfortunately, it can sometimes be difficult to find information on the different types of help that are available. You may need to be persistent in your enquiries. Your GP is likely to be a good source of information, but you should also talk to other carers. In this chapter, we discuss the kind of help that you will need, whether from family or from outside sources, such as the health service, local authority social services department and voluntary organisations.

FAMILY AND FRIENDS

Families are a very important source of practical help and support. Sometimes it is possible to share

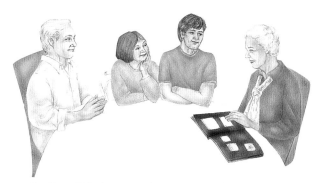

Families and friends are a very important source of help and support.

the responsibility of caring. A brother and sister, for example, might take it in turns to look after their father, or one member of the family may make a regular commitment to look after the sufferer while the carer has a break.

If, for various reasons, it is not possible to share the burden of care with other members of the family, friends may well be happy to offer practical help as well as a sympathetic ear. They may be able to sit with the sufferer while the carer goes out.

Your GP

Many other sources of practical support can be organised through your doctor. Health visitors, district nurses and community psychiatric nurses are usually part of the primary health care team attached to the GP's surgery. These nurses understand the practical difficulties of caring for a demented person at home. They can advise you whether any changes in health need to be reported to your doctor, and can teach you how best to overcome some of the practical problems of caring, such as bathing, eating problems, difficult behaviour, incontinence and giving medicines.

The district nurse can also provide help if the sufferer is frail and bedbound, or needs a great deal of assistance with bathing, dressing or putting to bed.

Occupational therapist

Your GP or hospital specialist can probably make arrangements for an occupational therapist to visit you. They can advise on and arrange for aids and adaptations at home; for example, hand rails, raised lavatory seats, bath seats, specially adapted cutlery and feeding aids, and

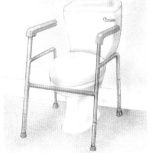

Handrails around a toilet promote security and stability.

gadgets to make dressing easier. They will also be able to advise you on eligibility for financial help to make major adaptations, such as installing a shower or wheelchair ramps.

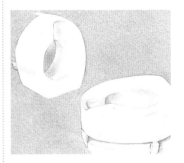

A raised toilet seat may be useful.

HELP IN THE HOME

Your local social services department may be able to arrange for a home-help to visit for several hours a week. They can provide practical help with housework, cleaning, laundry and shopping, and may also be able to assist with the personal care of the sufferer.

Meals-on-wheels services exist in most areas. They provide a hot meal delivered to the house on certain days of the week. This is useful for sufferers who are still able to live alone. Your local Citizens Advice Bureau or social services department will be able to give you more details.

FINANCIAL HELP

Caring for someone with dementia can be costly so it is important to

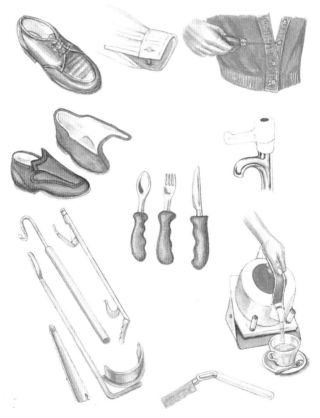

Household gadgets can help.

ensure that you are receiving all the financial help that's available. There are a number of benefits and allowances to which you and the sufferer may be entitled, such as the Attendance Allowance, Invalid Care Allowance and Disability Living Allowance. People with dementia may qualify for a discount on the Council Tax. The Citizens Advice Bureau or a social worker will be able to advise you on your eligibility and how to go about claiming these benefits. Some charities, such as the Alzheimer's Disease Society, may also be able to offer one-off grants to carers for specific purposes, if help cannot be obtained from other sources.

SHORT-TERM RELIEF

One very important way to obtain help with the care of a demented person is to arrange for them to be cared for away from home for part of each day. This provides short-term relief for the main caregiver and may enable you to continue working part-time if you want to. Your local social services department may be the best source of information on what is available in your area. Day centres, run by both local authorities and voluntary organisations, can provide recreational and social activities, lunch, and transport to and from home. Some day centres cater specifically for people with dementia. Psychogeriatric day hospitals, run by the health service, offer medical assessment, social activities and occupational therapy, but places are limited and usually short term.

Although day centres provide the most common form of relief care, it may also be possible to arrange for someone to come into

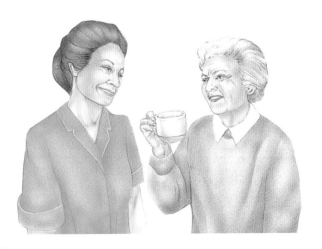

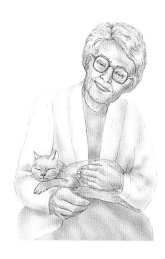

Pets can provide comfort.

time off. Private agencies can supply a care attendant or a nurse to look after the sufferer for longer periods, but this form of care is expensive.

If you want to go away on holiday or need to have a longer break from the burdens of caring, it may be possible to arrange residential care in a home or hospital. Some hospitals have a few beds reserved for respite care. This is care provided specifically to allow the carer a break. Social service departments run residential homes for frail elderly people, which may be able to offer relief care for short periods.

your home to care for the sufferer. Some voluntary agencies provide sitters for a few hours. Alternatively, local carers' support groups may arrange sitting services, with members taking it in turns, so everyone has the opportunity for time off.

Alternatively, you could use one of many private nursing and residential homes. Your GP or local social service office should be able to advise you what is available in your area.

KEY POINTS

✓ Practical and emotional support may come from family, friends, your GP, local carers' groups or your church (or other religious centre)

✓ Organisations that can help include the Citizens Advice Bureau, the Alzheimer's Disease Society and the social services

What can be done?

We have already described the way in which your doctor will try to find out what is causing the symptoms of mental deterioration. Should the cause prove to be a metabolic disturbance, a hormone deficiency or a vitamin B_{12} deficiency, your doctor will take steps to correct the problem and there is a very good chance that the symptoms will improve.

But what if the worst happens and it turns out that the symptoms are due to a progressive form of dementia, such as Alzheimer's disease? Can anything be done? Unfortunately, no treatment is yet available that can cure Alzheimer's disease. A few drugs have been given to sufferers experimentally in trials, to see whether they are effective at lessening the severity of the symptoms and slowing down the progression of the disease. Although some trials have

suggested that some patients may benefit from taking drugs, other trials with other groups of patients have failed to confirm the results. There is the disadvantage that some of these treatments carry a risk of quite serious side effects. Most of these drugs are not generally available because the hazards of taking them outweigh the potential benefits or because they are still at the experimental stage. However, two new drugs called donepezil (or Aricept) and rivastigmine (or Exelon) are now obtainable on prescription. Trials have shown that scores on some tests of mental function were slightly better in patients taking these drugs.

However, not all patients respond to these treatments and, even when improvements do occur, they may not be great enough to have a worthwhile effect on patients' symptoms or their day-to-day functioning.

After Alzheimer's disease, vascular dementia is the most common disease that causes dementia. It occurs when some of the small vessels that carry blood to the brain become blocked. The area of brain supplied by a blocked blood vessel dies through lack of oxygen. By the time symptoms are noticeable it is too late to try to unblock the vessel, but it is possible to try to prevent things getting worse.

Raised blood pressure is one reason why blood vessels tend to get blocked, and this can be treated safely and effectively with drugs.

Another possible cause of blood vessel blockage is that the blood flowing inside them tends to clot too readily. It has been found fairly recently that a low dose of a familiar drug – aspirin – is very effective in counteracting this tendency. A small daily dose of soluble aspirin is frequently advised for people whose blood is rather too liable to clot.

At the moment, most medical treatment of people suffering from dementia is aimed at reducing the problems that can make these people so difficult to look after. Effective treatments can be prescribed that will reduce restlessness and agitation and improve mood and sleep patterns. But these symptoms don't always require treatment with drugs and it may be better to tackle the problem in other ways.

BEHAVIOURAL PROBLEMS

As the disease progresses, sufferers may behave in ways that those caring for them find both distressing and difficult to cope with practically. People with dementia can sometimes behave in a very aggressive manner, becoming verbally abusive or even physically violent. They may over-react to what seems a slight setback and get frustrated, upset or angry. They may become agitated and restless, constantly moving around the house or wandering off for no apparent reason. Some sufferers may lose their normal inhibitions and start behaving in socially unacceptable ways, such as removing their clothes in front of other people.

If you are caring for someone with dementia, you may be able to deal with some of these behavioural problems by preventive measures. Take note of the sort of situations that are likely to give rise to such reactions and work out ways of avoiding them. Trying to maintain a calm, familiar and unstressful environment for the sufferer will help prevent outbursts of anger and distress.

You may be able to get advice on how best to deal with emotional and behavioural problems from a community psychiatric nurse. They provide support for people with mental health problems and their families. Your doctor should be able to arrange this for you.

If levels of distress, agitation and aggression are very high and do not respond to these simple measures, treatment with tranquillisers can be helpful. These drugs have a calming and sedative effect but they may produce unwanted side effects. They can be prescribed only by a doctor and must be used under close medical supervision.

TREATING DEPRESSION

It can sometimes be difficult to distinguish between the symptoms of severe depression and those of dementia. Correct diagnosis is very important because, unlike for dementia, effective drugs are available to treat severe depression. Sometimes people with dementia may become quite depressed. They cry frequently, appear withdrawn and are unable to enjoy anything.

Treatment with antidepressant drugs improves their mood, helps them to sleep, and may also lead to a reduction in behaviour problems. If you think the person for whom you are caring may be depressed, talk to your doctor, who may decide to get a specialist opinion from a psychiatrist or psychogeriatrician before prescribing treatment.

KEY POINTS

✓ There is no cure yet available for Alzheimer's disease

✓ Drugs designed to improve symptoms are becoming available

✓ The benefits of these new drugs seem to be modest

✓ Treatment with tranquillisers or antidepressants can reduce agitation and improve mood

Why did it happen?

Whenever a change in our lives is forced upon us, we all want to know the reason for it. So it is easy to understand why a diagnosis of dementia in a family member often leads people to try to find some event or factor that might have caused the disease.

If, for example, the symptoms of dementia first became noticeable after moving house, or in the months following retirement, it would be tempting to conclude that the stresses and life changes that accompanied these events were somehow to blame for the onset of the disease.

IT ISN'T YOUR FAULT

Some people go further than this and believe that they themselves may be to blame for what happened. They worry that something they did or failed to do may have caused the disease or made the symptoms worse. It's all too easy to find yourself thinking 'If only I'd taken her to see the doctor sooner', 'I should have taken more notice of the changes in him', or 'I wish I'd been more sympathetic'.

It is very important not to accuse yourself in this way. The symptoms of dementia appear so gradually that it is very hard to notice that something is wrong with someone whom you see every day. Friends and relatives who don't see the sufferer very often are in a much better position to recognise these gradual changes, and they're frequently the first to notice a deterioration.

THE CAUSES OF DEMENTIA

The causes of Alzheimer's disease are as yet unknown, although there are several theories that we discuss later in this chapter. A little more is known about vascular dementia. But, first, let's look at what does NOT cause the disease. A great deal of research is being carried out to learn more about dementia and why some individuals are susceptible to it. The results of this research show that many of the popular ideas about the causes of the disease are incorrect.

What NOT to blame

Underuse of the brain
Many people believe that mental faculties deteriorate if they're not used enough – this is sometimes known as the 'use it or lose it' theory. According to this view, old people are less likely to become demented if they remain mentally active and have lots of interests, but this is mistaken. Alzheimer's disease and other causes of dementia affect all sorts of people from all walks of life.

There are many good reasons to make efforts to keep your mind alert after retirement but doing so won't protect you from dementia.

Overuse of the brain
There is no evidence that 'thinking too much' can cause dementia – you cannot damage or wear out your brain by mental activity.

Stressful life events
Dementia is not caused by sudden changes or adverse events in daily life such as bereavement, divorce, moving house, being admitted to hospital or accidents, although such an event may sometimes bring a hidden dementia to light. The sufferer may have been able to cope previously, but a sudden change or a stressful experience may prove too much so that the symptoms of dementia become noticeable for the very first time. It may appear as if the event has caused the dementia but, in fact, the disease had already taken hold and the event only made it more obvious to other people.

Psychological problems
People who have suffered from anxiety or depression are sometimes thought to be more at risk of developing dementia, but there is no clear evidence that this is so. Depression is sometimes one of the symptoms in the early stages of dementia and this may be why it has mistakenly been regarded as a cause of the disease.

Alcohol
Alcohol, of course, affects brain function at least in a temporary way, so perhaps it is not surprising that many people believe that heavy or prolonged drinking can lead to a loss of brain cells. Sometimes brain damage does occur in malnourished alcoholics but this type of dementia is rare and is different from Alzheimer's disease or vascular dementia.

Smoking

It has been suggested that smoking may actually protect people against Alzheimer's disease, but as yet there is not a great deal of evidence to support this. However, smokers do seem to be more likely to develop another form of dementia known as vascular dementia.

Head injury

Everyday knocks, such as banging one's head on a kitchen cupboard, do not cause dementia, but people such as professional boxers who have been subjected to repeated severe blows to the head do sometimes develop a form of dementia. Experts argue about whether a single violent injury to the head, serious enough to result in loss of consciousness, increases the risk of Alzheimer's disease. If it does, the risk is not increased very much. Most people who survive a head injury will not get Alzheimer's disease.

Old age

Dementia is not caused by old age, and the majority of elderly people will not develop it. However, like almost every other illness, dementia is more likely to occur in older than in younger people.

MODERN THEORIES

There is a major research effort into the origin of Alzheimer's disease and explanations include genetic and environmental causes.

Genetics

In a small proportion of cases, all of whom develop the disease at an unusually early age, Alzheimer's disease runs strongly in their families. In some of these families, a defective gene located on chromosome 21 has been identified as the cause of the disease. This explanation, however, is the exception rather than the rule. Only a very small percentage of the total number of cases of Alzheimer's disease can be put down to this defective gene.

Recently, a genetic pre-disposition for the more common form of Alzheimer's disease, which affects older people, has been discovered. People who carry a particular form of the gene for apolipoprotein E are at increased risk. This gene contains the information that the body needs to make a protein that is important for the development and maintenance of the brain. There are three variants of this protein.

There is now good evidence that possessing one of these variants leads to an increase in the risk of developing Alzheimer's disease later in life. How this variant of apolipoprotein E acts to increase susceptibility to Alzheimer's disease is not yet understood.

Environmental causes

A very large number of possible environmental factors that might cause Alzheimer's disease have been investigated. These have included foreign travel, type of occupation, using chemicals, taking drugs and medicines, tea and coffee drinking, and malnutrition. There have also been studies to find out whether people who have had a surgical operation or a general anaesthetic or who have suffered from some other disease are more likely to develop Alzheimer's disease. The finger of suspicion does not point very strongly at any of these possibilities at present.

VASCULAR DEMENTIA

This form of dementia has its origin not in the nerve cells of the brain but in disease of the small blood vessels that carry oxygen and fuel to this organ. One very important factor that leads to disease of blood vessels is raised blood pressure. People whose blood pressure has been high for a number of years are more likely to develop vascular dementia.

Another factor that makes this type of dementia more likely is smoking cigarettes. This is because it increases the tendency of the blood to clot. The combination of disease of small blood vessels and blood that tends to clot too readily is dangerous. It is likely to lead to blockage of blood vessels and to damage to the areas of the brain supplied by the blocked vessels.

KEY POINTS

✓ In a few cases, people develop Alzheimer's disease because of a defective gene, but, in most cases, the cause of Alzheimer's disease is unknown

✓ One important cause of vascular dementia is raised blood pressure

The future

Alzheimer's disease, or any other form of dementia, is a personal tragedy for the sufferer and for those who love them and shoulder the burden of caring for them. It is a tragedy that is affecting more and more people.

Not so very long ago, doctors thought of Alzheimer's disease and other conditions that cause dementia as being quite rare. Today, everyone has heard of dementia and many have had the sad experience of looking after a close relative suffering from it. Why is this? One important reason is that the world's population is getting older.

THE AGEING POPULATION

At the beginning of the century, the average life expectancy of a new-born baby in the UK was about 50 years. Thanks to improved living conditions – better housing, better nutrition – and better medical care, an increasing proportion of each succeeding generation has survived into old age. The average life expectancy of a baby born today is now over 76 years. This improvement, together with the fact that people have been having smaller families, means that the population has been growing older. In 1951, only seven per cent of the population was aged 65 and over, but by 1996 this had grown to 18 per cent.

This ageing of the population means, of course, that there are many more cases of diseases that affect elderly people.

The population of the UK, and of almost every other country in the world, will continue to get older until well into the twenty-first century. We can predict that dementia will become an even bigger problem as time goes on. Countries in the developing world, such as Brazil, Kenya and Bangladesh, where populations are young and dementia still a rare condition, will soon be faced with the same problem.

RESEARCH INTO DEMENTIA

If you are looking after someone with dementia, you may feel very lonely. Perhaps it seems as if no one else cares much about what you are going through. This impression is quite wrong. There is a major medical research effort in all the countries of the Western World into discovering the causes of Alzheimer's disease and the other diseases that lead to dementia. Equally important, scientists are working hard to develop successful treatments for dementia.

Let us look at what has been achieved so far and what we hope will happen in the future. If progress seems slow, you must remember that even 20 years ago dementia wasn't thought to be a significant medical problem and it was low on the list of priorities for research. We knew very little about the condition then, so researchers had to start almost from scratch.

One of their first tasks was to find out how large the problem was. Epidemiologists – medical researchers who study the patterns of disease in the population – have carried out many surveys in different parts of the world and, as a result, we have a fairly accurate idea of how frequently dementia occurs. This information was crucial in drawing attention to the scale of the problem and how urgent it was to find out more about it. Some of these surveys also provided clues about the causes of some of the diseases that cause dementia. For example, the results of one study carried out in the UK hinted that Alzheimer's disease was more common in parts of the country where the drinking water contained small amounts of aluminium. Further studies failed, however, to confirm any link between aluminium and Alzheimer's disease, so this lead turned out to be a red herring.

In the laboratory, enormous strides have been made in understanding the processes that go on inside the nerve cells of the brains of people affected by Alzheimer's disease. We now know that a protein molecule whose normal function is to join one cell to its next door neighbour accumulates in abnormally large quantities in the brains of Alzheimer's sufferers. It appears that the cellular machinery that breaks down this protein when it is no longer needed fails. If we can find out why it fails it may be possible to do something about it.

Biochemists have discovered that levels of a chemical called acetylcholine are very low in some parts of the brains of people who have died from Alzheimer's disease. Acetylcholine is one of the chemical messengers in the brain; it allows one nerve cell to communicate with another. This discovery led to research to find a drug that would raise the levels of acetylcholine. It is hoped that replenishing stores of this chemical will partly restore brain function.

Geneticists are also working on the problem of dementia. An important discovery a few years ago was that in a small number of cases Alzheimer's disease is caused by a defective gene. If geneticists can now find out what the normal gene does, we may gain a better understanding of what goes wrong in the disease.

THE OUTLOOK

We don't yet know which of these lines of research will prove to be fruitful and which will turn out to be a blind alley. We can't predict where the next advance will come from, and it is important that investigation continues on a broad front. Finding out the causes of dementia and understanding what goes wrong inside the nerve cells of the brain is a very difficult task. Progress is slow and, if you are looking after someone with dementia, we must warn you that advances will probably come too late to help you personally.

Some people who know or look after a person with dementia decide to join one of the voluntary organisations mentioned earlier. These charities offer help and advice to sufferers and their families, and some also provide funding for scientists who are investigating the causes of dementia and trying to develop treatments. Individuals can help in a number of ways, whether taking part in fund-raising activities or volunteering to help with home sitting services, transport schemes or support groups. By getting involved in this sort of activity, people often feel that they have a chance to do something positive. It is one way in which good can come out of the tragedy that is dementia.

KEY POINTS

✓ People are tending to live for longer

✓ An ageing population means that cases of diseases that affect elderly people, including Alzheimer's disease, are on the increase

✓ There is a major medical research effort taking place to discover the causes of Alzheimer's disease and other diseases that lead to dementia

Further reading

DEMENTIA

Jane Brotchie (1998). *Caring for Someone who has Dementia.* Age Concern England.

Alan Jacques (1992). *Understanding Dementia,* 2nd edn. Churchill-Livingstone.

Nancy Mace and others (1992). *The 36 Hour Day: a family guide to caring at home for people with Alzheimer's disease and other confusional illnesses.* Age Concern and Hodder & Stoughton.

Robert Woods (1989). *Alzheimer's Disease: coping with a living death.* Souvenir Press.

MEMORY

Alan Baddeley (1996). *Your Memory,* 2nd edition. Prion.

Useful addresses

Age Concern England
Freepost (SW30375)
Ashburton
Devon TQ13 7ZZ
Tel: 0800 009966
(7 days; 7am–7pm)
Email: ace@ace.org.uk
Website: www.ace.org.uk

Age Concern Scotland
113 Rose Street
Edinburgh EH2 3DT
Tel: 0131 220 3345
Fax: 0131 220 2779
Website: www.ace.org.uk/scotland

Age Concern Northern Ireland
3 Lower Crescent
Belfast BT7 1NR
Helpline: 028 9023 3323
Tel: 028 9024 5729
Email: ageconcern.ni@btinternet.com

Age Concern Cymru
4th Floor
1 Cathedral Road
Cardiff CF1 9SD
Tel: 029 2037 1566
Fax: 029 2039 9562
Email: contact@accymru.demon.uk
Website: www.ace.org.uk/cymru

This is the largest charity providing services for elderly people in the UK. There are many local branches and groups, which provide a number of services, such as day care centres and support groups for carers (see your local telephone directory or get details from the address above). Fact sheets are available from local branches or the addresses above.

Alzheimer's Disease Society
Gordon House
10 Greencoat Place
London SW1P 1PH
Tel: 020 7306 0606
Helpline: 0845 300 0336 (Mon–Fri 8am–6pm)
Fax: 020 7306 0808
Email: info@alzheimers.org.uk
Website: www.alzheimers.org.uk

This Society aims to provide support to sufferers of dementia and their families. There are many local branches and groups (see your local telephone directory or get details from the address above). Information and advice sheets are available from the address above or from local branches or via the Society's Website.

Crossroads

England: 10 Regent Place
Rugby
Warwickshire CV1 2PN
Tel: 01788 573653
Fax: 01788 565498
Email:
crossroads.rugby@pipemedia.co.uk
Wales: Ground Floor
Unit 5, Coopers Yard
Curran Road
Cardiff CF1 5DF
Tel: 029 20222282
Fax: 029 20238258
Scotland: 24 George Square
Glasgow G2 1EG
Tel: 0141 226 3793
Fax: 0141 221 7130
Email: enquiries@crossroads-scot.k-web.com
Northern Ireland: 7 Regent Street
Newtownards
Co. Down BT23 4AB
Tel: 01247 814455
Fax: 01247 812112

Crossroads run care attendant schemes in partnership with health authorities and local social services. The aim is to bridge the gap left by other services. Trained care attendants come for several hours a week to give the carer a break. In most cases this service is free.

Carers National Association

20–25 Glasshouse Yard
London EC1A 4JT
Tel: 020 7490 8818
Fax: 020 7490 8824
Carers Line: 0808 808 7777 (Mon–Fri 10–12am and 2–4pm)
Website: www.carersuk.demon.co.uk

They aim to encourage carers to recognise their own needs, to provide information and advice, and to develop support for carers. Local branches organise a variety of activities to help carers, such as self-help support groups, social events and telephone helplines. The national office, at the address above, can put you in touch with a group or branch in your area. Leaflets and fact sheets are available from the address above or via the Website.

Citizens Advice Bureaux

CAB workers can offer advice and information on a wide range of issues, such as benefits, housing and family problems. To find your nearest CAB, look in your telephone directory or ask at your local library.

MIND – National Association for Mental Health
Granta House
15–19 Broadway
Stratford
London E15 4BQ
Tel: 020 8519 2122
Fax: 020 8522 1725
MIND Info' line:
Outside London: 0345 660163
Greater London: 020 8522 1728
Website: www.mind.org.uk

Mind Cymru
Third Floor
Quebec House
Castlebridge
Cowbridge Road East
Cardiff CF11 9AB
Telephone: 029 2039 5123
Fax: 029 2022 1189

This charity provides support for people with mental health problems, including dementia, and their families. There are many local groups, which may be able to offer a variety of services, such as day centres or support groups (see your local telephone directory or get details from the address above).

Useful links

Crossroads in Wirral
http://www.crossroads-wirral.org.uk

Carers National Association North of England
www.carersnorth.demon.co.uk

Information for carers on the Benefit Agency website
www.dss.gov.uk/ba/GBI/5a68151.htm

Local MIND associations
www.mind.org.uk/localmind/index.htm

Index

acetylcholine levels **54–5**
Age Concern **37**
ageing **5**
 – and dementia **51, 53–4**
 – and mental function **5–7**
aggression **24, 47**
agitation **47**
aids **42, 43**
alcohol and dementia **50**
allowances **44**
aluminium and dementia **54**
Alzheimer's disease
 – causes **25–6, 49**
 – the future **53–5**
 – in mixed dementia **28**
 – symptoms **23–5**
 – therapy **46**
 – see also dementia
Alzheimer's Disease Society **37,
    44, 57**
amyloid protein **26**
anger **37–8**
antidepressants **48**
anxiety **5, 24, 50**
apolipoprotein E **51**
appointments, forgetting **13, 15**
Aricept **46**
aspirin therapy **47**
Attendance Allowance **44**
bad language **20**
bags, losing **17**
behavioural changes **24, 47–8**
benefits **44**

blame, feeling **48, 50–2**
blood
 – clots **47**
 – pressure
   – high, and dementia **27, 46,
     52**
   – measurement **31**
 – supply to brain **26–7**
 – tests **33**
boxing and dementia **51**
brain
 – disease **19**
 – nerve cell changes **26, 54**
 – overuse **50**
 – scans **33–4**
 – underuse **50**
busy life **4–5**
calendars to help memory **15**
car parks, losing car in **18**
Carers National Association **37,
    57**
carers' support **36–7, 39, 41–5,
    55**
chest X–ray **33, 34**
chromosome 21 **51**
Citizens Advice Bureau **44, 58**
clinical psychologist **31–2**
communication problems **25**
community psychiatric nurses **42,
    47–9**
computed tomography scan
    33–4
concentration problems **20, 24–5**

conversation problems **25**
coping with forgetfulness **12–18**
Council Tax **44**
CT scan **33–4**
cupboards, labelling **17**
day centres **44**
dementia
  – case history **19–22**
  – causes **25–8, 49–50**
  – diagnosing **28, 29–34**
  – mixed **27–8**
  – research **54–5**
  – symptoms **23–5, 49**
  – what it is **23–9**
  – *see also* Alzheimer's disease;
    vascular dementia
depression **5, 28, 48, 50**
diabetes **5**
diaries to help memory **14, 15**
disability **5**
  – Living Allowance **44**
disorientation **24**
district nurses **42**
donepezil **46**
drugs
  – adverse reactions causing
    dementia **28, 31**
  – for dementia **46**
embarrassment about dementia
  38, 39, 47
emotional impact of dementia
  36–40, 47–8
energy loss **21**
environmental causes of
dementia **52**
epidemiology **54**
Exelon **46**
family, support from **37, 41–2**
financial help **43–4**
finding things **17–18**
forgetting things **3–4**
friends, support from **37, 41–2**
gardening, forgetting jobs **17**
genetic factors in dementia **26,
  51, 55**
geriatrician **32**
GP, support from **42**
grief **36**
guilt feeling **38–9**

head injuries causing dementia
  28, 51
health visitors **42**
hearing problems **5**
heart disease **5**
hereditary disease causing
dementia **28**
holidays
  – for carers **45**
  – lists for **16**
home help **43**
honesty
  – about dementia **39**
  – about memory **12–13, 14**
hormone imbalance causing
dementia **33, 46**
hospital respite care **45**
housework **43**
humour, keeping sense of **13**
illness **5**
infarction, brain **27**
information
  – recall **2–3, 4**
  – registering **2**
  – storage **2, 3, 23**
Invalid Care Allowance **44**
keys, finding **17**
labelling things **17**
laundry **43**
learning new things **5–6**
lists to help memory **14, 15–16,
  17**
loneliness **39**
loss, sense of **36–7**
lost, getting **21, 24**
meals-on-wheels **43**
medical history **30–1**
memory
  – ageing and **5–7**
  – aids **14**
  – how it works **2–3**
  – improvements for tasks
    16–17
  – interference with **4–5**
  – loss in dementia **23**
  – overload **4, 5–6**
  – prompts **14–16**
  – questionnaire **8–11**
  – types **3**

mental performance tests **31, 32, 46**

metabolic changes causing dementia **28, 46**

moodiness/mood swings **20, 24, 47**

names, remembering **1, 2, 6, 12–13, 18**

neurofibrillary tangles **26**

neurologist **32**

notes as reminders **14–15**

numbers, remembering **6**

nursing, private **45**

occupational therapists **42**

old age see ageing

personality changes **24**

positive attitude **12**

Post-it notes **15**

private agencies **44**

private nursing **45**

protein changes in brain **54**

psychiatric support **42**

psychiatrist **32**

psychogeriatric day hospitals **44**

psychogeriatrician **32**

psychological problems **50**

psychological support **37**

psychologist, clinical **31–2**

putting things away **17–18**

questionnaire on memory **8–11**

reaction times **5**

recall **2–3, 4, 22**

relief for carer
 – short–term **44–5**
 – see also support

reminders **14–15**

resentment **38–9**

residential care **39, 45**

respite care **45**

restlessness **47**

retirement **19**

rivastigmine **46**

role change in family **38**

self-assessment **12**

senile plaques **26**

shopping **20, 43**
 – lists **17, 14, 15**

sitting services **44**

skills, loss **21, 24–5**

sleep problems **47**

smoking and dementia **27, 51, 52**

social problems **47**

social worker help **44**

specialists in dementia **31–2**

spitefulness **24**

storage of information **2, 3**

strategies for coping **14**

stress
 – avoiding **47**
 – and dementia **50**

stroke **27**

support for carer **36–7, 39, 41–5, 55**
 – groups **37, 39**

tablet organisers **16**

tasks, memory improving **16–17**

telephone conversations **15**

temper outbursts **24**

tests and investigations **31, 32–4**

thyroid underactivity causing dementia **28**

toilet adaptations **42**

tranquillisers **48**

vascular dementia
 – causes **26–7, 49, 51, 52**
 – therapy **47**

verbal abuse **47**

violence **47**

visual problems **5**

vitamin B_{12} deficiency causing dementia **28, 46**

voluntary agencies **44, 55**

X-rays **33, 34**